N
S
2010

CON

INTRODUCTION	2
WELLBEING	3
STRESS	5
LOSS OF INTEREST IN SEX	10
IMPOTENCE	13
PREMATURE EJACULATION	17
DELAYED EJACULATION	19
INFERTILITY	20
PROSTATISM	22
TESTICULAR CANCER	24
HELP FROM THE EAST	25
MORE HELP	27
How to Use Herbal Remedies	28
How to Use Essential Oils	28
RESOURCES	29
PRACTITIONERS	30
SUPPLIERS	31

This book is presented as a collection of natural remedies and as an aid in understanding their use. It is not intended to replace or supersede professional consultation or treatment and no guarantee can be given as to the efficacy or appropriateness of a remedy in an individual case without professional advice.and no guarantee can be given as to the efficacy or appropriateness of a remedy in an individual case without professional advice.

INTRODUCTION

This booklet sets out to address some of the issues that commonly affect men's health and emotional security, especially in relation to sexual wellbeing.

Often misunderstood by men themselves, difficult to talk about and surrounded by taboo and misinformation, men's sexual vitality is in many cases left to chance, an ignored symptom of deeper unease. More often discussed and understood by women than men, real issues that affect many, many men become the subject of vague hints and suggestions at best and locker-room humour at worst.

The following pages, attempt to address concerns about sexual wellbeing with suggestions drawn from the fields of natural medicine. It is not a booklet about sexually transmitted diseases, and touches only briefly on the common medical conditions that affect men's sexual health, rather it is intended to concentrate on sexual energy, or the lack of it, and the factors that affect it and can improve it.

WELLBEING

Sexual anxiety, erectile dysfunction, premature ejaculation or infertility are all conditions that have an effect on many men's lives at some point or another.

In some cases there are clear medical reasons why symptoms are being experienced, and these will be touched on later, but for many men unease about, or disinclination towards, sex are indications that a toll is being taken on energy and resources in other parts of life.

What we may simply call our energy – or lack of it – the unquantifiable thing that makes us tick, is often referred to in Western natural medicine as the life force or 'vital force'. In Chinese and other Eastern medicines it is known as the 'qi'. By whatever name we call it the philosophy behind all natural medicines considers that it is this energy that holds the key to our body's health. When this energy is low, the body is susceptible to illness, whether physical or mental. In our fast-paced world the drains on our energy are many: cigarette smoking, alcohol, pollution, excess consumption of fat, salt and sugar in processed foods, inadequate exercise, lack of sleep and stress.

How each individual responds to these demands will differ from person to person, but it is common for a body lacking vitality and ease to be unable to express itself in a healthy sex life.

WHY DO WE IGNORE OUR WELLBEING?

So many men ignore the biological signs of illness both physical and psychological, that it would almost seem we have been socially conditioned to pay no attention to them.

It can come as little surprise that many men take no notice of symptoms of cancer of the testes or prostate because society still largely ignores men's health issues.

Emotional wellbeing is even harder to define and, so, very often the fatigue that warns against further activity and protects against exhaustion is pushed aside, either through necessity or through a misplaced belief that it is the 'heroic' thing to do. Whether physical or emotional, ignoring warning signs leads to the gradual breakdown of the body's natural activities.

It is a cliché to report that men find sharing their emotional problems difficult, but what results from it is born out in the figures for male suicide (the ratio for male to female suicides is 2:1) and heart disease (forty per cent of men who die in the 45-64 age group do so as the result of a coronary). The demands to succeed, provide for a family, achieve promotion and accumulate consumer goods all take their toll and manifest themselves in a myriad of different ways – raised blood pressure, ulcers, breathing problems and sexual unease.

If true wellbeing is to be achieved, then working to free ourselves of the stresses which cause our unease is essential to realizing the good health we all desire.

STRESS

Stress is a buzzword which everyone in the industrialized 21st Century world has some understanding of.

It is all too easy to dismiss our emotional or physical responses to a given situation as due to being 'stressed-out' or to excuse ourselves by saying we're 'just a bit stressed at the moment'. But if we remember that the word stress is derived from the word 'distress' we see that what we are describing is the body's suffering when tension has become unbearably high.

It is difficult to imagine life without stress and, in fact, a moderate level of stress may be important and beneficial: indeed, its very existence is crucial to our survival as a species. Early man's ability to survive depended on his ability to hunt and escape predators and the 'fight or flight' response is the body's way of coping with the threat of attack.

When danger threatens the body releases large amounts of the hormone adrenaline which instantly triggers the release of energy to the organs that are involved in defending the body: the heart pumps harder, breathing increases, blood vessels dilate, muscles tense, digestion slows, the testes are drawn up; all designed to make the body fight harder or flee quicker.

SURVIVAL RESPONSES IN THE MODERN WORLD

Although in modern life the need to flee from a sabre tooth tiger is rare, the reaction to any perceived challenge or threat is the same. The stresses in our lives are so abundant and continuous that our bodies end up in a permanent state of 'flight or fight' and instead of burning off energy generated for self-protection, it remains stagnant and we find ourselves in a continual state of tension.

Unfortunately, this unnatural state quickly leads to feelings of chronic stress and, over time, this exhausts us and we begin to experience physical and emotional symptoms. These may include headaches, indigestion, disturbed sleep, short-term memory loss, feelings of frustration, irritability, anger, depression and sexual problems, including erectile dysfunction (impotence).

Sources of stress may not be particularly dramatic or out-of-the-ordinary, in fact psychologists refer to them simply as 'life events'. They can be major upheavals – divorce, moving home, losing a job – or everyday situations – workplace problems, long journeys, even holidays – but if a succession of 'life events' follow one after another, or one particular 'event' remains constant the body doesn't have time to recover and the effects begin to be intense.

HEALTHY BALANCE

If a good sex life is an expression of the body's well-being, sexual problems may indicate that, somewhere, you are in distress. As discussed, a moderate amount of stress is inevitable, but if you are reading this booklet because you are experiencing sexual problems, thinking about your levels of stress and finding ways to counter the effects of stress on the physical and emotional levels may be the first step towards enhancing your levels of sexual vitality.

Aim for a balanced, healthy way of life that includes a nutritious diet with plenty of fruit and vegetables, regular exercise, adequate sleep most nights of the week, plenty of relaxation that restores sensitive nerves and heals the spirit. Try not to rely on things which mask the distress, but do nothing to solve the problem, for example smoking, comfort eating, excessive use of alcohol, too much coffee, tea or caffeinated drinks and abusing illegal drugs.

There are a number of natural remedies which have a long tradition of use to help relax a body suffering symptoms of stress and to help it recover. See which of the following seem best indicated.

HERBS

The following herbs all have a long standing reputation for treating the symptoms of anxiety and stress, and used in combination with herbs from some of the other sections in this booklet are an effective way of helping with problems of sexual health. For directions on how to take herbs and dosages, see the "How to Use Herbs" section towards the back of this booklet.

SKULLCAP *(Scutellaria lateriflora)*
Calming for many nervous conditions, it has a tonic effect on the central nervous system, so is ideal for nervous exhaustion, disturbed sleep or nervous stress following emotional upheaval or shock.

VERVAIN *(Verbena officinalis)*
An effective nerve tonic useful for nervous exhaustion, depression and irritability, particularly when there is sluggish digestion or a poor appetite. This is also the first herb of choice when anxiety is prevalent and should be considered for helping with premature ejaculation.

OATS *(Avena sativa)*
Porridge for breakfast is not just a nutritious meal! The herb is a good restorative nerve tonic for both physical and nervous weakness, ideal for depression and qi (energy) deficiency.

BALM *(Melissa officinalis)*
Sometimes referred to as the 'herbal hug' as it helps to lift the spirits and give you a sense of being cared for and protected. Lemon balm, an antidepressant herb, is also indicated when stress is affecting sleep or digestion. This herb is useful in any mix.

ESSENTIAL OILS

These may be diluted in a massage oil base to massage into the skin at a dilution of 2% (40 drops to 100ml), or a bath oil to add to the bath. As with herbs, oils are often more effective used in combination. For more information on directions see "How to Use Essential Oils" towards the end of this booklet.

BASIL

An excellent tonic for the nervous system and has a reviving and strengthening effect. It is useful when sexual problems are the result of tension, stress or overwork. Do not use basil for more than 6 weeks at a time.

BERGAMOT

Often thought as the oil for the angry young man. If your fuse is short, you are quick to temper and you tend to get all hot under the collar then this is the first oil of choice. It is useful in calming and cooling the nervous system.

CEDARWOOD

Indicated for chronic stress and anxiety. It has restorative properties and is useful for exhaustion, particularly if caused by prolonged stress or illness.

FLOWER REMEDIES

Flower remedies work on the emotional and mental level and are particularly good for symptoms of stress. Dr Bach 'discovered' 38 remedies for helping with various states of consciousness during the 1930's and they are very simple to use.

UNWIND BACH FLOWER REMEDY

Is a combination of his remedies specifically for helping to relax and – yes – unwind. Take four drops in water when needed. Also useful may be the Australian Bush Flower combination 'Calm and Clear'. Take seven drops when needed.

NUTRITIONAL SUPPLEMENTS

B COMPLEX

B complex vitamins help convert food into energy, essential when life gets especially busy. Vitamin B5 (pantothenic acid) is fundamental in many of the body's functions and will help support the adrenal system.

B vitamins may be found naturally in the following foods, or you can take a dietary supplement to boost your intake: yeast extract, whole grain cereals, pulses, green vegetables and dairy products.

OTHER IDEAS

Other measures may also be supportive. You might like to try reducing stress and tension by using complementary therapies, such as aromatherapy or massage. Relaxation techniques such as yoga or meditation may also be helpful or consider visiting a stress management counsellor who can help you talk about your problems and work out your own solutions.

When we begin to take control of the stresses in our lives, we generally begin to live a healthier life. We will often find that better food, more exercise and relaxation, less of the things that are bad for us, more of the things that are good begins to clear up specific symptoms. In the context of this booklet, that will hopefully mean that your anxiety about, or disinclination towards, sex will begin to change. If, however, you find that the particular concern you have is continuing despite instituting some of the above changes, the following sections will provide you with more information about what you can do, and remedies that may be helpful.

LOSS OF INTEREST IN SEX

This condition means that you lack interest in lovemaking or any intimate activity with a partner. This may well cause concern for you and your partner.

You may find that you rarely or never feel like having sex, that you have no desire and do not feel aroused, even in situations that would normally arouse you, or that you feel like having sex less often than your partner. Perhaps you will attempt to avoid love making altogether by making excuses to avoid situations where sex is likely or evading affectionate contact with a partner. You are not alone: according to a recent large survey about 15% of men aged 18-59 say they lack interest in sex (www.malehealth.co.uk).

Poor libido is one of the fastest growing sexual problems for men, probably due to the highly pressured lifestyles that many men now live and loss of interest in sex is, most often, caused by stress, depression, overwork or exhaustion. Again, finding ways to deal with your stress, getting enough sleep and taking regular exercise may be enough to help.

You may like to consider whether you have a different level of sexual desire from your partner which is causing tension and anxiety. In this case you will need to find ways to negotiate a compromise, perhaps with the help of a counsellor (see the Resources section for organisations that may be able to help).

Finally, you should consider whether there is a physical cause for your lack of interest. Desire for sex can be affected by hormonal imbalance and you should certainly get advice if you have other symptoms, such as a reduction in facial hair growth or a loss of body hair, shrinking testes or muscular weakness. These could be signs of testosterone deficiency so ask your GP for tests.

The following natural remedies may also be of use in improving interest in sex.

HERBS

It is important to be aware that herbs do not work instantaneously. When taking any mix you need to give them several weeks to work. The general rule of thumb is that for every year you have had a problem or condition a month of treatment may be required. However do not be surprised by their efficacy and potency!

DAMIANA *(Turnera diffusa)*
The most popular herb for helping a lack of interest in sex. It is a very versatile herb which has a reputation as an aphrodisiac but also is used as an antidepressant and helps combat chronic exhaustion and anxiety. Many also consider this herb to be the first choice in both premature ejaculation and impotence. Consider this herb as a starting point in any mix.

GINSENG *(Panax ginseng)*
One of a number of 'tonic' or adaptogenic herbs used in Chinese medicine to support the body during times of stress or illness. Ginseng is perhaps the best known of these and helps replenish qi and gives more energy. Research has identified compounds that are similar to sex hormones and this may be why it has a long standing reputation as an aphrodisiac. It is also said to help increase the motility and quantity of sperm and may be useful in preventing and treating testicular damage caused by environmental pollutants.

ASHWAGANDA *(Withania somnifera)*
Also known as 'Indian ginseng' and comes from the Ayurvedic tradition of tonic herbs. It has a reputation as an aphrodisiac, but, as well as helping to strengthen the nervous system it is known for aiding both impotence and infertility.

ESSENTIAL OILS

Oils that have a reputation as an aphrodisiac are the first to think of but it is often useful to mix these with oils for stress (see previous section) if this is indicated. They can be used in massage oil and applied in a clockwise motion between the belly button and the pubic bone. Repeat this massage over many weeks at regular intervals.

JASMINE
Often called the king of oils and has a reputation as an aphrodisiac particularly for men perhaps because it is so deeply relaxing and helps to dispel inhibitions.

YLANG YLANG
Is a flower used in Indonesia to cover the marital bed on the wedding night. It has been used for centuries as an aphrodisiac and to aid fertility. Balancing and calming to the nervous system it should be thought of first in any blend.

FLOWER REMEDIES

Many remedies may be of use, particularly to boost confidence and self esteem. However a good start is the combination Confidence and Power designed to give, believe it or not, confidence and power! The Australian Bush Remedy Sexuality Essence helps individuals to enjoy physical and emotional intimacy and renews passion and interest in relationships.

NUTRITION

RED FOODS
Have long been used to stimulate the senses and organs responsible for sexual activity. Carrots, beetroot, cayenne and tomatoes help boost many of the body's vital functions which can all contribute to an active sex life. Add more of these foods to your diet.

IMPOTENCE

Erectile Dysfunction (ED), to give impotence its proper name, describes the situation when a man's erection does not stay hard enough, long enough for him to have enjoyable sex.

The problem affects a surprising amount of men – up to one in ten in the UK (www.bbc.co.uk/health). In fact, most men will experience an erection problem at least once during their lives, which may be due to stress, exhaustion, too much alcohol (commonly called 'brewers droop'), or just not feeling like having sex. If the problem is persistent, however, it is an indication that there are underlying issues and it is important to begin to address these.

CAUSES

There are two main causes of ED: physical and psychological. For the vast majority of men, it is a physical problem and causes include:

- drinking too much alcohol which reduces testosterone levels, increases levels of the female hormone oestrogen and damages nerves leading to the penis
- the use of recreational drugs, like cannabis, which can lead to chronic impotence; diabetes (up to 25% of all diabetic men aged 30-34 are affected by ED, as are 75% of diabetic men aged 60-64 – www.malehealth.co.uk)
- high-blood pressure or atherosclerosis which can cause a shortage of blood to the penis
- spinal chord injury or surgery around the pelvis (such as prostate gland surgery) and the side-effects of prescription medication.

If any of the above are issues for you then a visit to the GP or other healthcare professional would be advised and there are a range of treatments available, both for ED and any underlying physical problems.

Even if the cause is physical, it is easy to become anxious or stressed about it and these feelings can quickly exacerbate the symptoms of ED. Stress and depression may also lead to Erectile Dysfunction, as might relationship problems, sexual boredom, or anxiety about sex or sexual orientation. As a makeshift test, if you can get an erection in some circumstances (during the night or on waking, for example), but not in others, the cause is likely to be psychological. The general advice about wellbeing is once again applicable: don't smoke (smoking is another major cause of damage to arteries leading to the penis), don't drink too much, eat well, sleep well, take regular exercise and make time for relaxation, but the following natural remedies may also be of benefit.

HERBS

Many of the herbs already mentioned may be appropriate for helping with ED. Ashwaganda and Damiana are specifically indicated but herbs for stress or anxiety may also be necessary. The following will help with blood flow to ensure adequate penile circulation.

GINKGO (*Ginkgo biloba*)
Used for periphery circulation and has a direct effect on the blood flow to the penile arteries and veins. It must be used for several weeks before it begins to take effect and should be continued for up to six months. If you are taking prescribed drugs check with a practitioner before using this herb.

HAWTHORN (*Crataegus oxyacanthoides*)
A herb that is used for increasing blood flow through the heart and thereby helping circulation throughout the body. If you are taking prescribed drugs check with a practitioner before using this herb

Using herbs in combination is normally advisable, as in cooking the final combination is usually greater than the sum of its parts!

ESSENTIAL OILS

JASMINE / YLANG YLANG
As mentioned in the previous section both of these should be considered as they have a relaxing and balancing effect on the nervous system. They could be combined with the following, Rosemary, oil and used in a massage oil and applied in a clockwise motion between the belly button and the pubic bone. Repeat this massage over many weeks at regular intervals.

ROSEMARY
An oil which helps with circulation and blood flow. It is stimulant and reviving to the nervous system and is helpful for debility and lack of energy.

FLOWER REMEDIES

OAK
Indicated for those who are normally strong but are weighed down by present circumstances. Although flower remedies principally affect emotional and mental states, they may also be of use where the physical reflects the emotional.

REVITALISE
A combination Bach Flower Remedy for anyone suffering from exhaustion and maybe useful to as short term help with lack of interest in sex or ED.

NUTRITION

L-ARGININE

Is an amino acid required for the production of nitric oxide. Nitric oxide is vital for the arteries supplying blood to the penis, as it allows them to relax and permit additional blood flow. (Viagra works through a mechanism that increases nitric acid production in these arteries). This is available as a food supplement.

PYCNOGENOL

Used in combination with L-Arginine, Pycnogenol (pine bark extract) can produce a significant improvement in ED. This is available as a food supplement in capsule form.

PREMATURE EJACULATION

U nlike Erectile Dysfunction, premature (or rapid) ejaculation is chiefly caused by psychological concerns.

There are physical causes – including diabetes, a tight foreskin or nervous system disorders – which would be best checked with your GP, but by far the most common causes are stress, anxiety about sex (perhaps due to fear of pregnancy or failing to perform adequately; nerves with a first or new partner; guilt during an affair) and lasting effects of previous unsatisfactory sexual experiences.

Ejaculation which occurs more quickly than a man or his partner would wish is the most common sexual dysfunction affecting men, and about one in three men of all ages suffer from premature ejaculation (www.malehealth.co.uk) at some stage in their sexual lives.

Many men can be helped to delay ejaculation, using self-help methods, but some may require the help of an expert practitioner. Some simple rules to follow include: making sure that you are free of anxiety during love-making if you can, learning to recognize the moment before you think you might ejaculate so that you can slow down or stop for a while and talking to your partner about the pressure you feel because of the problem. The Sexual Dysfunction Association produces leaflets that detail simple self-help techniques and can also put you in touch with qualified practitioners who may be able to help (see the Resources section).

These natural remedies may also be of use:

HERBS

Many of the herbs mentioned in previous sections may help, particularly herbs for stress. Damiana and Vervain are specific for treating premature ejaculation and should form the basis of a herbal mix.

FLOWER REMEDIES

Confidence and Power or Unwind Bach Flower Remedy combinations (both mentioned in previous sections), may both be useful but it may be necessary to choose a more specific individual Bach remedy depending on your emotional state.

DELAYED EJACULATION

As with premature ejaculation, delayed (or retarded) ejaculation is chiefly caused by psychological problems.

It is a difficulty which affects about one man in twenty (www.malehealth.co.uk) and is characterised by the inability to ejaculate, or a long delay before ejaculation, even though there is no problem with the man's erection and he feels aroused. It can be compounded by soreness due to prolonged stimulation in an effort to ejaculate.

If the problem is ongoing, it is worth having a check-up with your GP, or other healthcare professional, as the condition can be the side-effect of some antidepressant drugs; damage to the nerves; a physical injury or a hormone imbalance. If there is a deep seated anxiety about sex, perhaps as a result of a traumatic experience in childhood, ridicule from a previous sexual partner or a belief that sex is somehow dirty or immoral, delayed ejaculation may also become a problem. Counselling or therapy would be an appropriate course of action, and the addresses in the back of this booklet will be able to provide advice and put you in touch with a practitioner in your area.

In the main, however, exhaustion, tension and worry are principle causes, and any of the suggestions for relieving stress and anxiety given earlier in this booklet would be helpful.

INFERTILITY

Infertility is a widespread condition in which a couple is unable to produce children.

As many as one in six couples have a problem getting pregnant and male fertility is responsible in about half of these cases. The principle factor behind male infertility is the failure to produce enough healthy sperm. Many millions of sperm are ejaculated in each male orgasm, but only a few hundred make it to the fallopian tube where the woman's egg is fertilised. Any reduction in sperm count (the number of sperm ejaculated), any problem with their quality (if they are malformed, for instance), or with their motility (the sperm's ability to move spontaneously) reduces the chance of conception.

It is important not to worry unduly if your partner doesn't become pregnant straightaway – conception can sometimes take time even for the most fertile of couples – but visit your GP if you have been trying for a baby for more than a year without any luck. Talk to your partner before doing this; both of you will need to be checked out; infertility is a couple's problem and all good fertility clinics will want to see you together rather than one partner on their own.

If you suspect there are any physical problems – you are producing little or no semen or there is blood in it – or if you have been affected by inflammation in one or both testes (often caused by Mumps), enlarged veins around the testes, problems with the testes descending in early childhood, surgery in the pelvic area, ejaculation or erectile problems it will be worth visiting your GP immediately.

If there are no obvious physical problems, then stress, nervous anxiety or a low-state of general health are three major contributing factors to poor sperm health. Check out some of the following suggestions to maximise your fertility and ensure that you are in the best possible health to try for a baby.

HERBS

Professional help from a medical herbalist may be required to create a combination specific to you as an individual, however you could try combining Fleeceflower Root (below) with Ginseng and Ashwaganda (already mentioned).

FLEECEFLOWER ROOT *(Polygonum multiflorum)*

Another Chinese herb that is a vital tonic in herbal medicine. It is used to rebuild the strength and energy of the 'life force' and is said to promote longevity and virility. It has a reputation for treating infertility, by helping to increase the sperm count in men. It could be combined with Ginseng or Ashwaganda.

ESSENTIAL OILS

ROSE

As well as being well known for its benefits in treating infertility in women, using rose oil has been shown to increase the sperm count for men. Dilute in a base oil and massage in a circular motion into the area between the belly button and the pubic bone.

NUTRITION

ZINC

The prostate gland contains high amounts of zinc. When zinc levels fall too low, poor sperm production and reduced testosterone levels can result. Zinc supplementation may be useful, therefore, for male infertility. Smoking hinders zinc absorption so reducing or giving up is advisable.

PROSTATISM

Although not really within the confines of this booklet, many men, as they get older, suffer the embarrassing and irritating effects of the growth of their prostate gland.

The prostate produces secretions that are added to semen. Its normal size is approximately that of a walnut. It is situated at the base of the bladder and surrounds the urethra (the tube urine passes through). Once men reach their 40's the prostate gland begins to enlarge and, although for many men there are no problems, for others it can begin to cause discomfort. It is not entirely clear why this happens, but when it does, symptoms are likely to include: difficulty with passing urine; a weak stream that stops and starts; having to urinate frequently, often urgently, and dribbling after passing urine. Anxiety or embarrassment about these symptoms may cause other problems, such as loss of interest in sex or erectile dysfunction.

Although the most common cause of this problem is the non-cancerous condition Benign Prostatic Hyperplasia (BPH), which can be treated and managed fairly easily, similar symptoms occur in prostate cancer, so it is always worth checking with your GP in order to eliminate risk.

Benign enlargement of the prostate responds well to a natural approach. Try some of the following:

HERBS

SAW PALMETTO *(Serenoa serrulata)*
This herb has been proven to improve the signs and symptoms of an enlarged prostate by reducing the levels of a highly active form of testosterone, known as dihydrotestosterone which is thought to be largely responsible for enlargement of the prostate.

NETTLE ROOT *(Urtica dioica)*

Another herb which can combat prostate enlargement and reduce symptoms. It can be combined with saw palmetto to halt the growth of the prostate, and also with echinacea if there is any infection, horsetail if there is bleeding, cornsilk when there is pain and damiana if there is stress or sexual anxiety.

ESSENTIAL OILS

PINE

The antiseptic properties of pine have a beneficial effect on the whole urinary system and can help in prostatitis, especially when used in the bath. Try combining it with thyme.

THYME

One of the most important oils for treating the genito-urinary tract. These oils may also be combined in a base massage oil and massaged around the lower abdominal area and around the lower back a couple of times a day.

NUTRITION

PUMPKINSEED OIL

This is extremely rich in zinc, studies show that in conjunction with saw palmetto, pumpkin seed oil is very helpful in prostate health, and can benefit the bladder and urethra. You can eat raw pumpkin seeds on a regular basis or take pumpkin seed oil as a dietary supplement.

RED FOODS

Increase your intake of any red food, especially tomatoes, which contain a substance called lycopene, linked to a lower risk of prostate problems.

TESTICULAR CANCER

If men are reluctant to talk about their sexual health and well-being at the best of times, the problem becomes chronic with regards to testicular cancer.

Men are still dying from testicular cancer every year, yet, if it is detected early enough it is almost always curable. This booklet can clearly not recommend any course of treatment for testicular cancer, but it is vital that the message about testicular cancer gets across, and what better place than in a booklet about men's sexual health?

Testicular cancer is the most common form of cancer to affect men between the ages of 19 and 44 years old and its incidence has doubled over the past 20 years. Risk factors include family history and an undescended testis and symptoms may include a painless lump or swelling, a dull ache or enlargement in the testis.

The cure rate if the cancer is found early is 96%, so it is vital to examine yourself regularly (about once a month). After a warm bath or shower, hold your scrotum in the palm of your and use your fingers and thumb to gently roll each ball between them, looking for lumps, swelling, change in firmness or heaviness or any unusual shape. Remember, it is not unusual for one testis to be larger, or hang lower than the other so get used to what they feel like, or ask a health worker to show you. See your GP if you find anything unusual.

HELP FROM
THE EAST

In traditional Chinese Medicine, the kidneys are considered to be the root of all life.

The energy of the kidney is the link to millions of years of human evolution, enabling the transmission of genetic material. As well as maintaining our roots, the kidneys also enable healthy procreation and for that reason kidneys are the source of vitality, endurance, our instincts for survival and procreation. In Chinese Medicine the kidneys generate, store and activate the Essence or 'Jing'.

Jing is the original substance of an individual's life, it forms the basis of all tissues within the body and especially those of the human reproductive system. It governs all the developmental stages of life (birth, puberty, death) and is characterised by great stamina, ability to resist disease and sexual vitality. Impotence and sexual unease are characteristic of a loss of this essence and we need to conserve energy with sufficient rest and relaxation, by the avoidance of stimulants (e.g. caffeine) and chemicals and nourish it with good food and fresh air.

Many of the herbs mentioned in this booklet will help conserve and nourish our body's essence and you can either consult the individual sections or see the Men's Tonic recipe.

THE MEN'S TONIC BLEND

This combination of herbal tinctures was developed by the herbalist Dragana Vilinac to improve reproductive health and increase libido and fertility.

The formula is an excellent general tonic, and you will see that many of the herbs mentioned for individual problems in this booklet are combined here to provide help across the spectrum of male sexual health, as well as helping the body cope with stress and tension. 2mls of the tonic should be taken three times daily for a minimum of three months.

Damiana *(Turnera diffusa)*	2 parts
Ashwaganda *(Withania somnifera)*	2 parts
Ginseng *(Panax ginseng)*	2 parts
Fleeceflower *(Polygonum multiflorum)*	1.5 parts
Schisandra Fruit *(Schisandra chinensis)*	1.5 parts
Wolfberry Fruit *(Lyciium barbarum)*	1 part

For suppliers see page 31.

MORE HELP

Most natural therapists will work with your body's energy system to remove obstacles to health and vitality, and many stress-related conditions will then improve.

One outcome of visiting a practitioner is often an improvement to poor energy and libido. Also, practitioners are increasingly seeing people for specific sexual difficulties such as impotence and hormonal imbalances, and especially for fertility problems in both men and women.

Therapies that are particularly good at working to help deal with stress and improve general levels of energy and vitality include: aromatherapy, holistic massage, reflexology, counselling, naturopathy and shiatsu.

Therapies that are good at helping with specific problems such as impotence, hormonal imbalances and fertility problems include: acupuncture, herbalism and homoeopathy.

HOW TO USE HERBAL REMEDIES

You may need to take the herbs mentioned in this booklet for several weeks to establish a beneficial effect. You should review whether you need to continue taking the herbs after 3 months. Consider seeing a herbal practitioner for an individual prescription if your condition is not improving.

The herbs discussed in this booklet may be taken as a herbal tea or in tincture form. A tincture is an extraction of herbs using water and alcohol. They are a convenient way of taking herbal remedies because you just add a few drops to water.

DOSAGE

Herbal remedies are most often taken three times a day. Follow the directions on the packaging unless your practitioner advises otherwise.

SAFETY

Some prescribed drugs will interact with certain herbs and anyone taking medication should consult a practitioner before taking herbal remedies.

HOW TO USE ESSENTIAL OILS

Essential oils are the concentrated essence of a plant and must be diluted in a suitable vegetable oil, such as almond or sunflower oil, before use. To make a massage blend dilute 2% of combined essential oils into the base oil (20 drops is approximately 1ml; so add 40 drops to 100ml of base oil). Similarly, essential oils must be pre-diluted in a vegetable oil base before adding to the bath. To make a bath oil 4% of essential oils may be used. Essential oils should never be taken internally without the advice of a suitably qualified medical practitioner.

RESOURCES

The following organisations may be able to provide further help:

Relate
Herbert Gray College
Little Church Street
Rugby
Warwickshire CV21 3AP
Telephone: 01788 573241
www.relate.org.uk

Institute of Psychosexual Medicine
12 Chandos Street
Cavendish Square
London W1G 9DR
Telephone: 020 7580 0631
www.ipm.org.uk

The Sexual Dysfunction Association
Windmill Place Business Centre
2-4 Windmill Lane
Southall
Middlesex UB2 4NJ
Telephone: 0870 7743571
www.sda.uk.net

The Prostate Cancer Charity
3 Angel Walk
Hammersmith
London W6 9HX
Telephone: 0845 300 8383
www.prostate-cancer.org.uk

Men's Health Forum
News, information and discussion on men's health policy:
www.menshealthforum.org.uk
www.malehealth.co.uk

PRACTITIONERS

To find an practitioner in your area contact:

HOMŒOPATHY

The Society of Homeopaths
11 Brookfield,
Duncan Close,
Moulton Park,
Northampton
NN3 6WL
Tel: 0845 450 6611
www.homeopathy-soh.org

Alliance of Registered Homeopaths
Millbrook,
Millbrook Hill,
Nutley,
East Sussex
TN22 3PJ
Tel: 08700 736339
www.a-r-h.org

AROMATHERAPY

The Aromatherapy Consortium
PO Box 6522
Desborough
Kettering
Northants NN14 2YX
0870 774 3477
www.aromatherapycouncil.co.uk

HERBALISM

The National Institute of Medical Herbalists
56 Longbrook Street,
Exeter,
Devon
EX4 6AH
Tel: 01392 426022
www.nimh.org.uk

NUTRITION

British Association for Nutritional Therapy (BANT)
27 Old Gloucester Street,
London
WC1N 3XX
Tel: 0870 606 1284
www.bant.org.uk

SUPPLIERS

NEAL'S YARD REMEDIES

To find your nearest shop contact 01747 834634
Mail order: 0845 262 3145
www.nealsyardremedies.com
- Bach flower essences, herbs, tinctures, essential oils, homœopathic remedies, supplements.
- Therapy rooms offering a wide range of therapies for physical and emotional issues.

AINSWORTH'S HOMŒOPATHIC PHARMACY

36 New Cavendish Street,
London
W1G 8UF
Tel: 020 7935 5330
www.ainsworths.com

HELIOS HOMŒOPATHY

89-97 CAM DEN ROAD,
TUNBRIDGE WELLS,
KENT
TN1 2QR
WWW.HELIOS.CO.UK
TEL: 01892 537254